Sciatica Pain Relief –
Your Ultimate Solution to Living a
Pain-Free Life

Sciatica Pain Management Techniques and Relief Solutions

Disclaimer

"Sciatica Pain Relief – Your Ultimate Solution to Living a Pain-Free Life: Sciatica Pain Management Techniques and Relief Solutions"

What This Book Has For You

Are you experiencing a very uncomfortable pain in your back? Does it make it difficult for you to move around easily and live a normal life? If so, you could be suffering from sciatica pain. Sciatica Pain Relief is the ultimate book that will help you open up your world! Everything you want to learn about why you keep experiencing this unwanted pain is discussed and described in detail in this book to help you live a pain-free life. It also discloses all the options you have at your disposal to prevent the pain from happening again.

It is easy to understand and implement the techniques and methods discussed in this book because it is easy to read, no fluff, straight to the point, and gives you information that you are looking for. The book includes detailed instructions along with illustrations to help you understand your condition even better. You will find all of the following topics covered in this book:

- A detailed understanding of what sciatica is, detailed sciatica nerve anatomy, about sciatica nerve and different types of sciatica nerve pain.
- The common causes of sciatica pain and the reasons why you could be a victim too.
- The common symptoms of sciatica pain –covered all the possible warning signs that you should not ignore in order to diagnose sciatica pain. The chapter also includes details about symptoms associated with different sciatic nerves.
- Details about the non-surgical treatment and alternative methods that could be used to relieve sciatica pain. Some of these can be done at home to ease down the pain.
- The different exercises and how physical activity can help relieve sciatica pain – different exercises are discussed and even explained step by step to help you perform it.
- Introduction of yoga in your daily life and its benefits to treat sciatica symptoms –stretch exercise are also explained step by step to help you perform them.
- Surgical options are also discussed in detail in this book.

This eBook goes inside sciatica in an easy-to-understand way. Anyone can use the information and take advantage from it. So open up to a new life by using all this information and getting rid of sciatica pain for life!

So get started now. Good luck!

Contents

Chapter 1 – Understanding Sciatica

Before reading about what sciatica is all about and how you can avoid this pain, let us first understand sciatica in definition. This chapter will cover the simple definition, the sciatica nerve anatomy, and the different types of sciatica nerve pain in detail.

Read it all!

What Is Sciatica Pain – Learning from the Definition

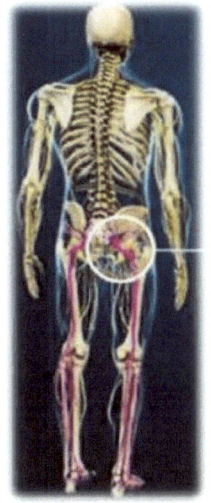

The term sciatica is a term used to describe pain affecting the hip, back and outer side of the leg. Sciatica is often caused by compression of spinal nerve root in the lower back, often owing to degeneration of an intervertebral disc. In addition to the pain, the compression of spinal nerve root can also lead to weakness, numbness and even tingling. However, the pain usually originates in the lower back area and in severe cases travels through the hips and down the large sciatic nerve in the outer side of the legs.

Sciatica (pronounced as sigh-at-ih-kah) is a symptom and not a medical diagnosis in and of itself. It is characterized as a symptom of various underlying medical conditions, including spinal stenosis, degenerative disc disease, and lumbar herniated disc.

In order to characterize sciatica pain, one or few of the following mentioned symptoms are often taken into consideration:

1. Regular pain in one leg or one side of the hip (rarely can occur in both legs and both hips as well).
2. Leg pain that also hints feelings like tingling, burning, or searing.
3. Pain that becomes worse while moving and sitting.
4. Numbness, weakness and difficulty in moving the foot or leg.
5. Unbearable, sharp pain that may make it difficult to walk, sit or stand up.

Sciatica pain is not the same experience for all. The pain can greatly vary from irritating and infrequent to incapacitating and constant. Specific symptoms of sciatica can vary when it comes to severity and location, depending upon the individual reasons causing sciatica pain.

While sciatica symptoms can be potentially debilitating and painful, it is rare that permanent damage to the sciatic nerve will result.

Sciatica and the Sciatic Nerve

As mentioned earlier, the symptoms of sciatica occur when the sciatic nerve is compressed in the lumbar spine or when it is irritated. It is actually a very large part of the sciatic nerve since the nerve itself is the largest one in the body and is also comprised of individual nerve roots that branch out from the lower back and spine.

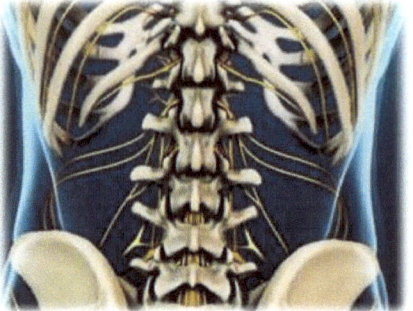

-   The sciatic nerve is located in the lower back at lumbar spine segment 3 (also known as L3).
-   The sciatic nerve begins from the lower back and moves down all the way to the back of each leg passing from the buttocks.
-   The sciatic nerve branch out in portions in each of the legs to innervate specific parts – the toes, foot, calf, and thigh

Symptoms of sciatica pain – pain in the leg, tingling, numbness, weakness, burning sensation and possibly symptoms that radiate into the foot –greatly depends on which area of the nerve is pinched. For instance, if the lumbar segment – which is also known as L5 –nerve is pinched, it can lead to weakness and numbness in the ankle as well as in the toe.

The Sciatica Pain Course

Sciatica is more common than you think. Even youngsters these days are complaining about back and leg pain. However, the incidence of this type of pain increases once you reach in middle-age. While it is becoming common these days –thanks to our sedentary lifestyles, busy schedules, desk jobs and wrong physical posture of walking and sitting–in youngsters now, it rarely occurred before the age of 20. The probability of experiencing sciatica pain is at its highest in the 50s before it starts declining.

Some people also confuse sciatica pain with pain caused by injuries. Often, this is not true. Sciatica pain symptoms often develop over a course of time and are not a result of injuries. Some people who experience sciatica pain tend to get better with time – in few weeks or months –and find relief in pain without the need of surgical sciatica treatment. However, it is important for them to take the non-surgical pain relief methods into account to get rid of the symptoms quickly. On the other hand, for other people the lower back and leg pain can be debilitating and severe and requires surgical treatment immediately.

As mentioned above, some of the sciatica symptoms can be worse and may require immediate medical and even surgical intervention. Such symptoms include progressive neurological symptoms and can lead to bladder or bowel dysfunction, leg weakness, etc.

Because sciatica is associated with an underlying disease or medical condition, the treatment of the pain is also focused on the same underlying causes that lead to the sciatica symptoms, such as herniated disc or spinal stenosis. At first, non-surgical treatment are considered and recommended for self-care and relief from sciatica pain, but for intractable or severe dysfunction and pain, and patients are often advised to consider surgery for pain relief.

Sciatica Nerve Anatomy

The sciatic nerve is the longest and largest single nerve designed naturally within the human body. The nerve is as big and round as a man's thumb at its largest point.

If the lower spine experiences any trouble it often affects one of the nerves that is located in that area and causes pain. The sciatic nerve, since it is the largest one, supplies strength and sensation to the legs along with their reflexes. It connects the outer part of the thigh with the spinal cord along with the muscles in the feet, lower leg, and back of the thighs. When sciatic nerve is damaged or affected, it can immediately cause pain and feeling of tingling and numbness in the foot, ankle, toes or the entire leg.

The Anatomy of Sciatic Nerve: The Combination

There are total five nerves that make up the sciatic nerve. It is formed on both the left and right sides of the lower spine by combining the 4th and 5th lumbar nerves while the first three nerves are located in the sacral spine. All of these nerves are located between two vertebral segments and are named according to the segments that are above it. For instance:

- The nerve present between the 4th and 5th lumbar segment is known as the L4 nerve root. Similarly, the nerve that exists between the L5 and sacral segment 1 is named as L5.
- The three nerves that emerge from the sacral spine are named as S1, S2 and S3 nerves.

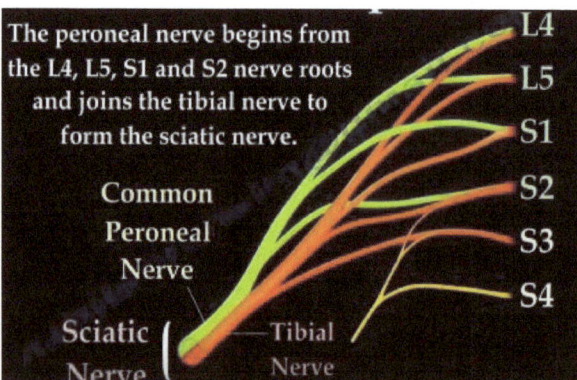

The group of 5 nerves together in the rear as well as the front of the piriformis muscle combines to become one large nerve, which is called the sciatic nerve. This major nerve then goes down right to the foot in each leg and branch out to provide sensory and motor functions to different regions in the leg.

The sciatic nerves further divides into two different nerves at the back of the knee in the lower thigh region. These nerves are known as the peroneal and tibial nerves. These nerves are further innervates to travel in different regions of the lower part of your leg.

- **Peroneal nerves –**this nerve move down sideways in a lateral manner along the outer part of the knee and travels towards the upper foot.
- **Tibial nerves –** this nerve move down in the same direction behind the knee and travel towards the feet and innervate the sole and heel of your foot.

Since different nerves follow different pathways to travel down to the foot, symptoms that a patient experiences could also be different and may present in different regions of the foot or leg. Everything depends on which part of the nerve is affected.

Types of Sciatic Nerve Pain

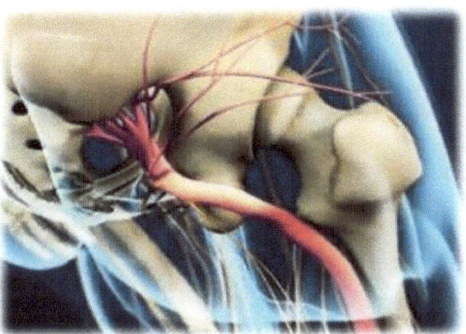

All of the sciatica symptoms, including nerve pain, tingling, numbness, and weakness –are variable. There is no one definition of what type of pain you will feel. Sciatic nerve pain include symptoms primarily in the thigh and buttock, pain traveling from thigh to the calf, and sometimes all the way to the toes.

The pain and individual symptoms can usually be traced according to the region where the nerve is affected. Some of the different types of pain and typical symptoms include:

- **Sciatica from L4 Nerve Root:** Symptoms from this level in the lower part of the spine usually cause numbness and/or pain in the foot and lower leg area. Weakness may cause hindrance in flexing the feet.
- **Sciatica from L5 Nerve Root:** When this segment is affected, a patient may experience pain and weakness in the extension of the ankle as well as the toes.
- **Sciatica from S1 Nerve Root:** At this level, which is the bottom part of the spine, the patient may experience numbness and/or pain to the outer part of the food. Again, the pain can cause difficulty in raising your feet off the ground.

While these are some common symptoms that a patient may experience, symptoms can greatly vary depending on various factors, such as the characteristics and degree of specific pathology as well as the unique anatomical variances.

Chapter 2 –What Causes Sciatica Pain: 5 Common Causes You Should Know About

As mentioned in the beginning of this book, sciatica itself is not a disease. This pain is often associated with the underlying medical cause that leads to a number of sciatica symptoms. Even the treatment for sciatica pain is focused on treating the root cause and medical condition so that you get rid of the pain permanently.

These underlying medical reasons will be discussed in this chapter in detail. These are the 5 most common causes that lead to sciatica pain. These problems are often related to your lower back area and causes severe pain, numbness and even tingling in your lower body. Get yourself checked to find out if you are suffering any of the following medical issues for your sciatica pain.

Read it till the end.

Lumbar Herniated Disc

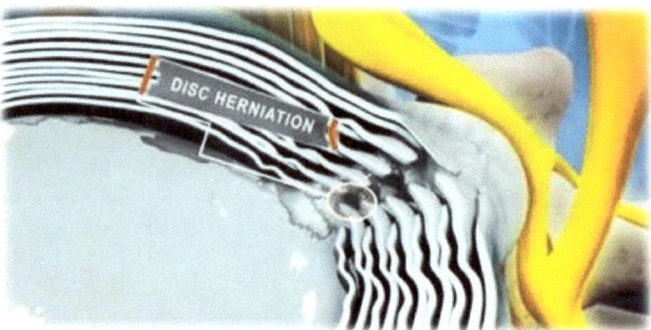

This medical problem occurs when the inner soft core of the disc herniates or leaks out through the fibrous core. The leakage causes irritation to the contiguous nerve root.

Some familiar names of lumbar herniated disc are ruptured disc, slipped disc, protruding disc, bulging disc, or a pinched nerve. Sciatica is a very common symptom that you might experience if you have a lumbar herniated disc.

As the disc breaks down or degenerates, the inner core leaks out. The soft core within the outer core is right under the spinal nerve root. Therefore, when the leakage takes place in this area, the pressure is directly on the spinal nerve.

Other common symptoms of lumbar herniated disc symptoms include:

1. Sciatica—leg pain is the most common of all, which may or may not occur without lower back pain. If you have lumbar herniated disc, the leg pain will typically be a lot worse than the pain in the lower back.
2. Weakness in the legs. You may face difficulty while walking.
3. Feeling of numbness or tingling in the leg as well as the foot. Again, this could make walking difficult.
4. Pain in the lower back area along with pain in the buttock.
5. Loss of bowel or bladder control (rare). This is, however, a declaration that your medical condition is serious than you think. Also, it could also be an indication towards a serious medical issue known as cauda equina syndrome.

Treatment for Lumbar Herniated Disc

In majority cases, treatment can help a patient feel better within about 6 weeks. The pain and other symptoms will slowly and gradually fade away, making the patient feel healthier.

While keeping an eye on the symptoms and their response, a number of non-surgical treatments can help alleviate pain and facilitate permanent or long-term healing as well. Some of the most common treatments for lumbar herniated disc (non-surgical) include:

- Ice and/or heat therapy
- Physical therapy
- Chiropractic/osteopathic manipulation (also known as manual manipulation)
- Oral steroids (e.g. methyprednisoloneor prednisone)
- An epidural
- Non-steroidal anti-inflammatory drugs

After taking these non-surgical treatments, if the pain persists even after six weeks duration, it is appropriate to consider microdiscectomyas your next more viable option.

Lumbar Herniated Disc Surgery

Next comes the option to go under the knife to get rid of the pain. This surgery helps take the pressure off the nerve root and provide a more suitable healing environment for the disc. During the surgery, the small part of the disc that is degenerating and is also pushing against the nerve and damaging it may also be removed if required. In majority of the cases, the intervertebral disc is not touched during the surgery.

If you are dealing with an experienced surgeon, the success rate of this surgery is as high as 95 percent!

Recurrence of Disc Herniation

There is a 10 percent change for patients to experience another discherniation in the same local, even after surgery. However, it is easier to judge if you are experiencing a recurrence because the symptoms would probably start showing in the postoperative period (which means the first three months). A recurrence may also happen after years. Fortunately, another microdiscectomy can be carried out to take care of another disc herniation case.

In case of multiple recurrence of lumbar disc herniation, a lumbar fusion surgery can be considered. This surgery stops the disc level motion and removes all of the disc material as well.

Degenerative Disc Disease (DDD)

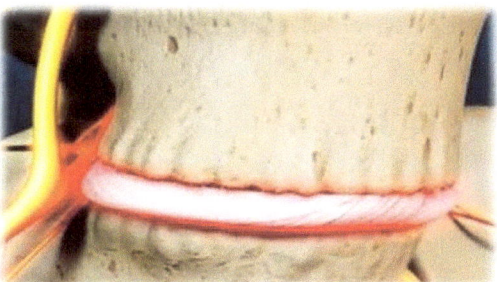

Degenerative Disc Disease is something that mostly comes as a part of aging. It is a natural process that cannot be prevented. This process causes one or more discs to degenerate in the lower back, which can irate a nerve root and lead to sciatica pain.

The DDD is diagnosed when a degenerated or weak disc leads to excessive micro-motion and expose out the inflammatory proteins from inside the disc. This irritates the nerve root in the region and cause pain and discomfort. The disease occurs in the lower back, or lumbar spine, and refers to all symptoms that are a result of compromised disc.

In addition to the age factor, genetic component may also be a major reason people suffer DDD. However, majority cases are said to be multi-factorial. There could be a traumatic cause behind the symptoms while in some cases it could just be due to simple wear and tear.

However, it is very rare to find out that such a disease is a result of a traumatic accident that caused injuries. In most cases, DDD is diagnosed when the disc faces a low-level injury that tends to grow and progress with time.

Since there's no supply to the blood, in case of an injury, it is not possible for the disc to repair itself like other tissues can. Other than this, insignificant injuries to the disc may also lead to degenerative cascade, in which the disc is completely damaged after some time.

While the name may strike really hard – degenerate disc disease –it is more common than you think. As mentioned above, the DDD dramatic label is unavoidable in cases where both age and genetics are playing their cards against you. More than 30% of people between the ages of 30 and 50 years experience some level of disc space degeneration, although everyone will not experience symptoms or pain or will require proper diagnosis. In fact, for patients who are in their 60s are rarely exceptions to some degree of disc degeneration.

Causes of Lumbar DDD

If you are experiencing sciatica or lower back pain, it could be because of lumbar degenerative disc disease. The chances increase if you age between 30-50 years old and have a family history of the disease. Other than these factors, the most common causes behind Lumbar DDD are as follows:

1. **Inflammation** –Since the protein present in between the disc space is exposed and starts irritating the surrounding nerves (including both the large and smaller nerves present within the disc space), which causes nerve pinching and causes pain in the lower back, buttocks and legs.
2. **Abnormal Micro-Motion Instability** – There is an outer protection ring on each disc known as the annulus fibrosus. When the protein is exposed, these rings are worn down and fail to absorb stress on the spine and cause the pain to travel down all the way to the feet.

When inflammatory proteins are excessively combined with the micro-motion, it can cause an ongoing, severe low back pain. Fortunately, DDD can be treated. For some people, the pain naturally starts fading away after a while. For others, it could continue progressing and can get worse, although it is more uncommon.

Degenerative Disc Disease Symptoms

Patients suffering DDD will experience bearable but continuous in the lower back area and thighs. While the pain and discomfort is tolerable, it can intensity occasionally and can go on like that for days.

Just like any other lower back disease, the symptoms for this one can also vary based on different factors, some of the most common ones are listed below.

1. Feeling pain right in the center of the lower back, which may intensify to travel to the legs and hips as well.
2. Continuous pain in the lower back (tolerable), which may last for more than a month or six weeks.
3. Experiencing a painful sensation in the lower back, as opposed to burning or searing pain, which radiates.
4. Experiencing pain while making certain moves, such as sitting, getting up from a low surface, twisting, bending and lifting.
5. Experiencing pain that gets worse in the sitting position, when the discs experience a heavier load as opposed to the standing, laying down, and walking position. Long time standing may also increase the pain just like lifting a heavy object or bending in awkward position would do.
6. Experience symptoms that are severe, including tingling and numbness in the legs. This could lead to problems in walking well.
7. Experiencing pain or symptoms from minimal motions, which eventually weakens the disc.

Other than the pain in the lower back part from degenerative disc disease, other symptoms may also include:

- The exposure of proteins can create inflammation between the disc space, which can eventually lead to low back pain radiating into the upper back thighs and buttocks area.
- The same pain can also travel down towards the foot from the back of the legs.
- The lumbar DDD can also play a role in the development of lumbar osteoarthritis and/or lumbar stenosis, as well as progression in the pain as well as lower back conditions.
- Other disease DDD could lead to includes to a lumbar herniated disc.

Lumbar Degenerative Disc Disease Treatments

Fortunately, lumbar degenerative disc disease can be treated for most people without the need of surgeries. Conservative care consisting of medication and alternative therapies can be used to control pain and inflammation. This can be achieved through steroid medications delivered through epidural injections or through oral methods. Other methods to achieve similar health goals are exercise and physical therapy.

While surgical options are also available to treat lumbar degenerative disc disease, they are only considered when a patient fails to achieve relief from pain or the condition for more than six months of non-surgical care or the condition is progressing while performing daily chores or activities.

The constant pain, as well as the intensity and frequency of the flares, can be avoided by following a number of non-surgical, conservative options.

Common Nonsurgical Treatment for Degenerative Disc Disease

Some of the best and most successful conservative treatment methods usually include some combination of the following:

- **Physical Therapy and Exercise** —Including an exercise program is important for the overall health as well as relieving the pain caused by DDD. In fact, exercise is considered a crucial part for almost all types of treatment program that help fight off conditions like lumbar degenerative disc disease. As far as the exercise program is concerned, several components of exercises and physical therapies should be includes. These are:
  - o **Hamstrings Stretching**—If the muscles in the hamstring area and down the back are tightened, it can cause stress on the back and can worsen the pain caused by lumbar DDD.
  - o **Back Strengthening Exercise**— While choosing the right exercises, it is important to keep the focus on your back and lower body muscles to avoid the pain. Exercises such as dynamic lumbar stabilization, where patients are taught to find their 'natural spine' and practice it. This is the most comfortable position for their spine and maintaining the right posture is what helps them get relief from the pain.
  - o **Low-Impact Aerobic Conditioning** – Exercises such as biking, swimming, walking are some of the low-impact exercises that you can follow in addition to following proper flow of nutrition to achieve optimal health. This is not only healthy for the overall system but also helps flow blood and nutrient to spine structure, and relieves pain by relieving pressure on the disc.

Experiencing constant pain in the back creates urge of resting more for the patient. However, it is not advised to rest for more than a day or two if you are already diagnosed with DDD. Engaging into activities and putting your spine to use in the right postures and moves is the best way to relief pain.

- **Icing and Heating Methods**–Both icing and heating methods can be used to increase range of motion and flexibility in the joints and stiff muscles. Application of heat can be done with the help of heating pads while ice packs can be used on the affected areas to calm down sore muscles. Icing also creates numbness in the area to control the extreme painful flares.
- **Medications** –There are a number of medications that play a role in relieving pain and provide comprehensive treatment for DDD. The common medications used are:
  - **Prescription medications with stronger impact** –medications including muscle relaxants, oral steroids, or narcotic medications for pain relieve are often given to manage the episodes of intense pain for temporary purpose. However, some patients may show long-term benefits in pain relief and muscle soreness by taking epidural steroid injections.
  - **Non-steroidal anti-inflammatory**–(e.g. COX-2 inhibitors, naproxen, and ibuprofen)and other medicines that help in relieving pain include acetaminophen are some medicines that help patients get rid of the pain and feel good enough to participate in daily chores and activities.

While the above mentioned medicines are great for some patients, not all of them are suitable for all patients. It is important that you consider your case individually and discuss with your doctor the important factors and side effects that would preclude taking the medicines.

Bottom Line

Postures are extremely important when it comes to managing back pain. If you are into some desk job, sitting for 8-10 long hours straight can make the situation worse. Therefore, it is important that you pay attention to your sitting posture. And if it is difficult for you to be so focused on the way you are sitting, you can get a Bael Wellness Seat Cushion that will do the job for you. This is designed especially for people experiencing sciatica pain and all you have to do is just place this cushion on your seat. The special design of this seat cushion will ensure your spine is in the perfect posture at all times.

Isthmic Spondylolisthesis

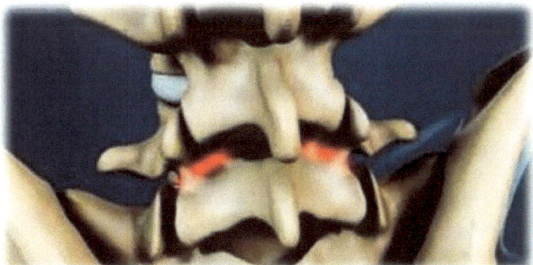

This condition is often experienced when an insignificant stress fracture allows one vertebral body to slip and adjust in front of the other vertebral body. For instance, if the L5 vertebra slips forward over the S1 vertebra, it will be known as Isthmic Spondylolisthesis.

The fracture occurs when a number of disc space collapse and allow the vertebral slipping forward. The nerve in between the vertebral body gets pinched, which causes sciatica pain. The stress on the bone is often caused by the fracture that takes place in the parsinterarticularies – which is a small piece of bone. This condition is more common in with younger individuals (kids around 5 to 8 years old), for majority people, symptoms will only start showing during the adulthood.

According to a survey, it was revealed that around 5% to 7% population has either spondylolisthesis (slipped vertebral body) or fracture in the pars interarticularies (small piece of bone). However, in majority cases, no symptoms are recognizable. In fact, estimations have been made based on facts and research that more than 80% of the people with the condition will never be able to experience any symptoms of spondylolisthesis. And for people where this condition will become symptomatic, a very small percentage of people will experience it in severity where surgical treatments are needed.

The Causes of Spondylolisthesis

Pars interarticularis are actually Latin words, which mean 'bridge between two joints'. This bridge is responsible for connecting the facet joint above to the one below. This bridge is a very small and thin bone and does not have proper blood circulation. This is one of the main reasons why it is so susceptible and sensitive to stress fractures. The fracture of this bridge is also possible without a vertebral slip. However, the fracture itself is called a spondylolysis. Other than the connecting bridge, the pars interarticularis are also sometimes called the isthmus.

At the fracture of this bone, a patient may not feel stress or any kind of pain in the area. In short, there are no symptoms and you wouldn't even know if the bone has fractured. Trauma is not a common reason behind the fracture. It is usually the cumulative stress that leads to this fracture.

The most common area of the spine where isthmic spondylolisthesis occur includes the L5-S1 levels. These are located at the tail of the lumbar spine. It is rarely above this level however, in case the fracture is caused in the upper levels, it is often caused by the trauma instead of cumulative stress.

The bone fracture has never been recorded in a newborn baby and therefore isn't considered a congenital problem. However, the fracture that occurs during childhood is likely to progress with time in adolescent individuals. It is very rare for grown up individuals to experience a progressive curve in the condition if they have developed it as grownups.

The Grading of Spondylisthesis

In order to diagnose the slippage, experts refer to the x-ray reports. However, the diagnosis is also done to measure the severity of the condition. This is easier with side-view x-rays to find out the real picture of the factor. Later, it is graded according to the 1-4 scale of grading.

The slippage or fracture is measured according to the number of upper vertebral body slips forwards on the lower vertebral body. The grading system is mentioned below:

Grade 1	25% or less of vertebral body has slipped forward
Grade 2	26% - 50%
Grade 3	51% - 75%
Grade 4	76% - 100%

The severity of the condition increases as the grading system moves towards a bigger number.

Another condition – although very rare –spondyloptosis may also occur. In this condition, the L5 vertebral body slips off the sacrum and goes right into the pelvis. The good news is that majority of the slips cases fall into either grade 1 or grade 2 scales only. Even though there are no symptoms, but in case the condition becomes symptomatic, it is possible to treat them without surgical procedures.

Isthmic Spondylolisthesis Symptoms

For patients who experience the symptoms of the condition, some common ones include:

1. Pain in the lower back. The pain is often a deep ache and can get severe with time.
2. Painful flares that keeps on radiating into the hips as well as the back of the thighs. This pain is also referred to as radicular pain.
3. Pain that gets worse while walking, standing or by involving into any activities that require backward bending position.
4. Pain that gets calm in the sitting position, especially if your body is in the reclining posture.
5. Pain that radiates into the foot from all the way down the knee.
6. Feeling of weakness and tiredness in the legs.

7. Numbness in the legs, especially after a brief walking session.

Other than the symptoms mentioned above, most patients with this condition may also experience tighter hamstring muscle. It is a large muscle that is located on the back side of the thigh. Tightness caused in this muscle can cause discomfort in moving and running and may even cause difficult for patients to bend and touch their toes.

Symptoms for Grade 2, Grade 3, Grade 4 Spondylolisthesis

Patients who are diagnosed with grade 2 or higher spondylolisthesis may experience more symptoms in addition to the ones mentioned above. This is because the worse the condition would be diagnosed, the deformity in the lower back will be more recognizable, especially if the slip also caused in a very vertical angle. These include:

1. The patient will also experience physical changes and may appear to have a larger abdomen and a shorter trunk.
2. Patients will also have comparatively larger vertical pelvis and lordosis.
3. The hamstrings of patients diagnosed with grade 2 or higher spondylolisthesis will often are very tight, which leads to problems in moving around and even a causes a waddling gait.

In rare cases, patients may also complain about experiencing symptoms associated with cauda equina syndrome. These symptoms will include: progressive weakness or numbness in the legs, uncomfortable sensation in the altered saddle area between the legs, and difficulty in controlling bladder or bowel movement.

If you are experiencing such symptoms, it is important that the patient seeks for urgent medical attention.

Isthmic Spondylolisthesis during Adolescence

Isthmic spondylolisthesis is considered a common reason that causes back pain and lower-back pain and discomfort during adolescence.

The research and facts encourage us to suspect that spondylolysis, the fracture in the bridge-bone is what leads to spondylolisthesis, is very common in young athletes to experience this in young age. Young ones who are passionate about sports and involve in activities and games that repeatedly require hyperextension of the lower back often leads to spondylolisthesis. Gymnastics are also considered one of the major activities that cause this condition.

Some of the most common symptoms (if it is symptomatic) include leg and/or back pain that causes discomfort at movement and therefore limit the activity level of the patient. In cases of higher grade of slips (grade 2 or higher), the patient may even notice a sway back or forward curve (which is unnatural) in their lower back area. During adolescence, development of paralysis and/or neurological problems is also possible; however, such cases are extremely rare.

Treatment for Spondylolisthesis During Adolescence

It is very common for adolescents who are into a lot of physical activities and sports to develop back pain over time. This pain is progressive and can show more symptoms with time if the patient continues to participate in the activity and/or sports. If you are diagnosed with spondylolisthesis on x-ray, it is often advised that you refrain from intense physical activity and sports until you get relief from the pain.

As far as the treatment for spondylolisthesis in adolescents is considered, there are various non-surgical treatment options that can be used for managing the pain. Some of the common ones include:

1. **Pain Medication** –acetaminophen and NSAID's are good options. However, it is highly recommended that you check with your doctor before taking any medication for pain relief.
2. **Heat and/or Ice Therapy** – To relieve pain, these are some great options too. Use heating pads or ice packs on the affected area and relieve flare-ups. This, however, is only a temporary relief and pain may return after the effects are gone.
3. **Physical Therapy** –While sports and intense physical activity – including gymnastics – are not recommended in case you are diagnosed with spondylolisthesis, physical therapy that helps the muscles loosen up can be useful in relieving the pain. This specifically applies to stretching the hamstring muscles. Since the condition causes this major leg muscle to tighten up, it can create additional stress across the fracture and the disc. Therefore, incorporating a few stretching exercises for the hamstring can break the cycle of pain and provide you with flexibility as well as relief from pain.

Lumbar Spinal Stenosis

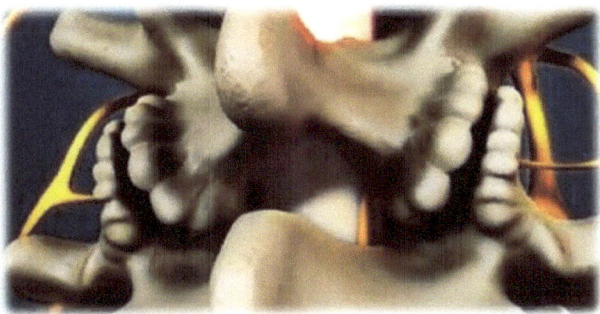

The next cause that leads to sciatica pain is the lumbar spinal stenosis. This condition occurs when the spinal canal narrows down and pinches the sciatica nerve. Lumbar spinal stenosis does not have to be associated with an injury or accident in all cases. In fact, in most cases it comes with natural aging and spinal canal narrowing is a very common condition in people above 60 years.

One or few of the symptoms often lead to lumbar spinal stenosis: overgrown soft tissues, enlarged facet joints, and a bulging disc placing that puts pressure on the nerve roots and causes you to bear sciatica pain.

As we begin aging, it causes changes in our spine. Unfortunately, these changes are not the positive ones and often lead to a degeneration of bones (vertebrae), ligaments (connective tissues), muscles, and disk that as a combination make up the spinal column. These changes are also the major causes behind spinal disc stenosis and thus, this condition is associated with aging.

Stenosis is a word that actually comes from a Greek word, which means 'choking'. This is the perfect way to describe the condition of the nerves when the spinal canal narrows down. In addition to aging, other factors that could narrow down the spinal canal include degenerative conditions such as degenerative spondylolisthesis and/or osteoarthritis. When the narrowing causes the spinal nerves to get squished and choked, it leads to lumbar spinal stenosis and often causes symptoms like lower back pain and leg pain.

More symptoms are described below.

Symptoms of Lumbar Spinal Stenosis Symptoms

One of the most easily recognizable symptoms is the increase in the severity of pain in the legs, especially when you are walking. This could actually become challenging when it comes to following an activity level or simply doing simple household chores and other work-related tasks.

Patients who are diagnosed with spinal stenosis do not experience any symptoms and are typically comfortable when at rest but it is almost impossible to move one step without the leg pain. Once the patients get back to the sitting position or get back into rest, pain relief can immediately be achieved. However, this relief is only temporary and comes with different postures.

Other than leg pain, there are no standard symptoms for all patients. In fact, the number of symptoms and their severity, both will vary and fluctuate during the course. Certain periods are rather comfortable with less symptoms and less severity while at other times, the duration, severity and number of symptoms can be very uncomfortable.

The type of symptoms you will be experience will actually dictate the type of treatment that will be suitable in your case. For instance, if the condition gets unbearable, doctors might suggest you to get surgical treatment while in other cases, conservative or non-surgical treatments can be taken to relief pain and get rid of the lumbar spinal stenosis.

The symptoms may not get severe in the beginning but keeps on growing with time. Majority of the patients are above 50 years old and symptoms can come and go.

Some of the most common symptoms of lumbar stenosis may include:

1. Leg pain and lower back pain (sciatica pain)
2. Numbness, weakness, or tingling that radiates from the lower back and travel to the legs all the way down from the buttocks.
3. Leg pain that grows while walking (claudication).

As the symptoms for the lumbar spinal stenosis worsen, they may get hard to bear. A survey estimates that more than 400,000 Americans suffer from lower back and/or leg pain due to lumbar spinal stenosis and most of these adults are above 50 years of age.

Treatment for Lumbar Spinal Stenosis

There are a number of non-surgical treatment options available for lumbar stenosis. The most common treatment include some or a combination of the following non-invasive treatment options.

- **Activity Modification:** As far as a comfortable position is concerned, patients feel better while at rest. However, during activity, flexed forward is the most comfortable position for the patient. For most patients, it is easier to ease discomfort and leg pain when walking by leaning forward on a shopping cart, walker, or a cane.
- **Physical Exercise:** Exercise will be treated as a non-invasive treatment method for patients diagnosed with lumbar spinal stenosis. Your doctor or spine specialist may suggest flexion exercises that help you alleviate the pain. These exercises will be forward bending, which is a comfortable position for the patient. Back exercises are also a part of the targeted program as these exercises help in alleviating the sciatica pain that is often caused by lumbar spinal stenosis. These exercises are a combination of strengthening and stretching exercises that mainly focus on:

- o Stretching the major muscle on the back to hold the spine in extension
- o Strengthening the muscles by forward bending and bringing the spine into flexion position.
- **Epidural Injections:** These injections are given on the basis of an out-patient and usually take around 30 minutes for the procedure to finish. The physician guides a needle into the spinal canal (right between the sac and lamina, which is the actual epidural space). Once the needle reaches the right location, the epidural solution is slowly injected. Steroids are used by the epidural injections as an anti-inflammatory agent and often include a fast-acting pain killer and local anesthetic for temporary relief from pain.
- **Non-steroidal Anti-Inflammatory Drugs (NSAIDs):** One of the most common components associated with the spinal stenosis is inflammation. Since that's the case, anti-inflammatory drugs are often prescribed to the patient for temporary relief from the pain. Drugs such as naproxen, ibuprofen, or Cox-2 inhibitors are given to the patients as an effective non-surgical treatment for patients diagnosed with lumbar spinal stenosis.

Surgical Options for Lumbar Spinal Stenosis

Surgery in such cases is always considered as a last resort. In cases where symptoms are not severe, it is always recommended to consider the simpler, non-surgical methods first. However, if you are diagnosed with lumbar spinal stenosis and the symptoms have forced you to reduce your everyday activities to an unacceptable level and you haven't really achieved any solution through the non-invasive methods to relieve symptoms, it is time to consider your surgery options.

For a majority of patients, opting for a lumbar spinal stenosis surgery is a choice for their lifestyle. For instance:

- If patients are willing to give up on a number of activities, they may want to take up surgery to relieve pain on a long-term basis.
- If patients are not functioning low to an unacceptable level, taken the risk for undergoing a surgery does not make any sense.

In addition, for the majority part, the chances of completely recovering from the condition and its symptoms are too low to consider this as a viable option. In fact, cases have been recorded where patients complain going for multiple spinal stenosis surgeries to get rid of pain.

Lumbar Laminectomy

For patients considering surgical treatment for lumbar spinal stenosis, lumbar laminectomy is their most suitable option. It is the most common form of surgery with the highest success rate. Some evidences show success rate to be as high as 80 percent. Fortunately, in majority of the lumbar decompression surgery, people recover to the level where they are able to return to their previous pain-free and active lifestyle.

Other Surgical Options

Although laminectomy is one of the most popular and recommended surgery option for spinal stenosis, other methods of surgical options include:

1. Laminotomy
2. Foraminotomy
3. Interspinous process spacer
4. Microendoscopic decompression.

Bottom Line

While there are a number of surgical options available, it is still recommended that you consider the alternative treatment methods first.

Piriformis Syndrome

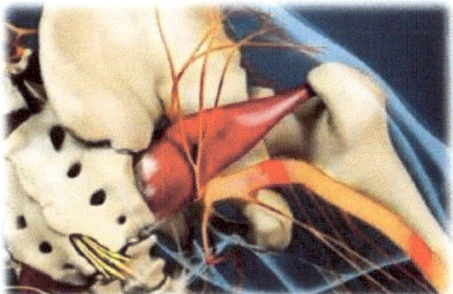

Piriformis syndrome is associated with the piriformis muscle located in the buttock region. In this condition, the sciatic nerve gets irritated as it runs down under the buttock region. The piriformis muscle pinches or irritates the nerve root, which also consists the sciatic nerve, and therefore can lead to sciatic pain.

The pain isn't really sciatica if you refer to the clinical definition of sciatica since it does not root to the spine. However, the leg pain caused by the condition is just like sciatica and so are the other symptoms.

When the piriformis muscle spasms and cause pain in the buttock, it also pinches or suffocates the sciatic nerve that runs down to the leg and foot and leads to sciatic nerve pain. The pain in the foot and the back of the leg can also cause tingling and numbness.

What You Need to Know About the Piriformis Muscle

While the role of piriformis muscle is quite significant, it isn't a very major muscle in the body. In fact, it is a small one located in the buttock.

The piriformis muscle:

1. Begins from the lower spine region and goes all the way to the upper surface of the thighbone and connects with it. The thighbone is also known as thighbone.
2. The function of the piriformis muscle is to assist in turning the foot and leg outward as well as rotating the hip.
3. The muscle runs diagonally while the sciatic nerve runs vertically right under the muscle. In some cases, the nerve also runs through the muscle and can cause higher intensity of pain.

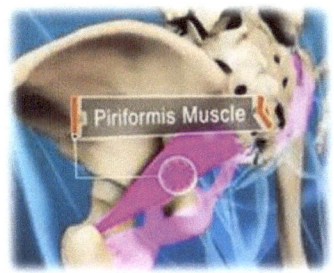

Piriformis Syndrome and Its Causes

There are no clear reasons behind the piriformis syndrome. However, some suspected causes include:

- You can experience spasm in the piriformis muscle for various reasons – including irritation caused within the muscle or irritation that is affecting a nearby structure such as your hip or the sacroiliac joint.
- The syndrome may also occur due to swelling in the piriformis muscle. This is often a cause of spasm or injury.
- Tightening of the piriformis muscle may also lead to piriformis syndrome. Tightness can also be caused by muscle spasm or injury.
- If the piriformis muscle or the surrounding area starts bleeding, it can also lead to piriformis syndrome.

One or few of the symptoms mentioned above can affect the piriformis muscle and lead to sciatica pain as well as pain in the back of the legs and buttock area. This will also have an effect on the adjacent sciatic nerve and can cause tingling, pain, or numbness in the foot, calf, or back of the thigh.

Symptoms for Piriformis Syndrome

Patients who are diagnosed with piriformis syndrome often only complain about sciatica-like pain and acute tenderness near your hip region. The sciatica pain often runs down starting from the buttock region to the foot and can be very uncomfortable for some patients.

Some of the most common symptoms include:

1. A dull but slightly uncomfortable ache in the hip region.
2. Pain that runs down in the thigh (usually at the back part), foot and calf. This is the pain that is referred to as sciatica-like pain.
3. Increase in pain in the legs and buttock region when walking up inclines or staircase.
4. The hip join causes pain when you try to increase the range of motion.
5. Pain caused by prolong hours of sitting.

It is easier to figure out the symptoms of sciatica mainly because the pain tends to get worse with different postures such as prolonged walking, sitting or running and instantly gets better as soon as you lie on your back and give your body some rest.

Non-Surgical Treatment and Therapy for Piriformis Syndrome

As far as the non-surgical treatment methods and therapy is concerned, the main focus will be on stretching exercises. When a patient indulges into a number of stretching exercises for the hip extensors, hamstrings, and piriformis, it may greatly help in controlling the symptoms and relieving sciatic nerve pain. Also, performing stretching exercises helps the patient experience the range of motion once again and without feeling intense pain.

Piriformis Stretching Exercises

For stretching exercises, there are multiple ways to stretch your piriformis muscle without causing further trouble. Two of the most common stretching exercises include:

1. Lie on your back with your knees bend and feet flat on the floor. In the same posture, pull your right knee towards your chest and bring it as close as you can. Use your left hand to grasp your knee and pull it towards your left shoulder. When you reach the peak stretch point, hold and let your body stretch. Relax and let go and put your foot back to the ground. Now repeat with your left knee in the same manner.
2. Get back in the same posture and lie down on your back with your knees bent. Now raise your right foot from the ground and place the ankle over the left leg knee. Now raise your left leg and pull it towards your chest. This will cause the stretch to happen on the entire buttock region. Hold for a minute or two and release. Repeat the same process with your left leg.

You may not be able to perform these exercises in the best possible manner in the beginning due to the pain and hurdles in twisting your hip bone. So try holding the stretch for at least 5 seconds in the beginning. Once you get hold of the posture and flexibility, go ahead and increase the stretching time and take it up to 30 seconds on each side.

It is also advisable that you perform this task 3 times in a day for better results.

Hamstring Stretches

As mentioned earlier, hamstring is a large muscle located at the back of thighs. Stretching these muscles through exercise can greatly help you alleviate sciatic pain and other symptoms. There are several ways to stretch the hamstrings.

- Place two similar chairs facing each other at a distance. Sit down on one chair, raise your leg and place the heel on the other chair. You can start with your right leg. Lean forward and bend the hips until you start feeling a gentle stretch in your hamstring muscle. Hold into that position. Release and do it with the other leg.
- For the second hamstring stretch exercise, lie on your back and keep your legs stretched and straight. Place a towel under your right tight and lift up the leg. Do not put the weight or pressure on your hands. Lift the leg by yourself. Keep your leg straight and stretched and bring it closer down towards your body until you feel a mild stretch on the hamstring muscle. Hold for a few second and release. Repeat with the other leg to complete the routine.

Again, you might face difficulty in holding the stretch in the beginning. So start with 5 seconds and gradually increase time up to 30 seconds for each pose. Follow this hamstring stretch routine three times in a day and see great results.

Other Physical Therapies for Piriformis Syndrome

Other than the basic stretching exercises, a detailed exercise and physical therapy program can be developed to suit the individual situation and condition of each patient. These physical therapies include:

- Range of motion exercises
- Deep massage
- Ice and heat therapy

Medications for sciatica pain associated with piriformis muscles include:

- Piriformis injection: corticosteroid or local anesthetic injection.
- Botox injection: botulinum toxin as a weakening agent.

Last but not the least, in addition to non-surgical methods and medication, the application of electrical stimulation can also help you achieve relieve from the pain. These electrical stimulations are known as interferential current stimulator (IFC) and transcutaneous electrical nerve stimulation (TENS) that helps in reducing muscle spasm and also alleviates pain associated with piriformis syndrome.

Other Causes of Sciatica

In addition to the 5 most common causes of sciatica mentioned above, here are some more conditions that can lead to sciatica pain. These include:

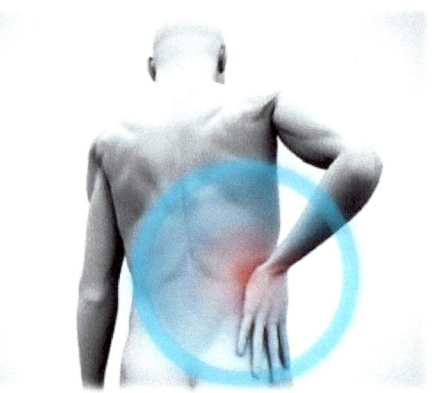

- **Pregnancy:** Pregnancy requires a woman's body to go through several changes, including weight gain. While the whole shift of hormones and gravity is going on, it is very common for women to experience sciatica pain during pregnancy.
- **Muscle Strain:** In a number of cases, inflammation liked with muscle strain can also suffocate the sciatica nerve by putting pressure on it. This can also lead to severe sciatica pain.
- **Scar Tissue:** Scar tissues also have the tendency to compress your nerve root and eventually the sciatica nerve. This can cause lower back pain and tingling in the legs, which are symptoms of sciatica pain.
- **Infection:** While infections are extremely rare, if you have an infection in the lower back part of body, it can also lead to sciatica by causing you pain.
- **Spinal Tumor –** Again, this is also very rare but if you are diagnosed with a spinal tumor, it can also have an impact on the nerve root located in the lower back. This can also cause you to suffer sciatica pain.

Now that we have seen all the common causes in detail and also learned about how each of the cause can be taken care of, let's move on to sciatica symptoms and how you can deal with the condition itself.

Chapter 3 – Sciatica Symptoms – The Warning Signs

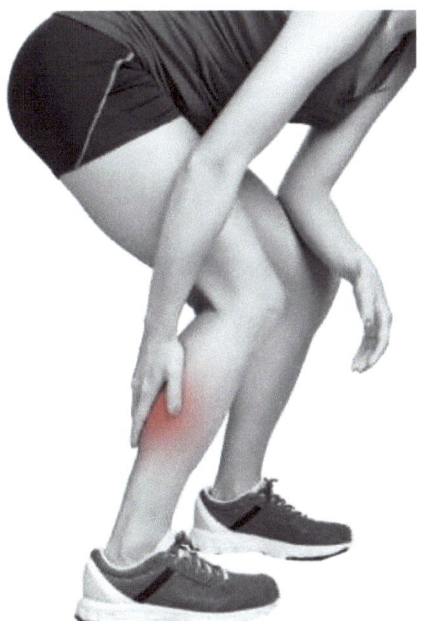

Some people might find sciatica totally unbearable because of the severe pain. For others, the symptoms could be very insignificant and hard to judge. While sciatica symptoms are irritating in all cases, their frequency is what creates the whole difference. All in all, the condition has the tendency to get worse and debilitating if not taken care of at the right time.

For people going through sciatica symptoms, low-back pain is a very common one. You might experience only pain in your lower back while at other times it comes along with leg pain as well. However, for patients who also experience leg pain usually complain about more severe pain in their legs as compared to their lower back pain. People also describe experiencing symptoms as a burning pain, searing pain, or electrical shocks running down the leg.

What You Need to Watch Out For

It is important to be aware of the most common symptoms so that it is easy to identify your condition. The following is a list of pains and conditions that you need to watch out for sciatica:

- Pain in the lower back – not extremely severe but uncomfortable.
- Pain that travels down the legs – if experienced a t all –and which can be much severer as compared to the back pain.
- Constant pain in either left or right buttock, which continues along the path where the nerve root or sciatic nerve is located. These regions include the backside of the thighs and all the way to the legs and foot.
- Experiencing pain that is either very dull or extremely sharp.
- Some people even complain about experiencing pain that gives them a 'pin and needle' sensation, weakness or numbness, and sometimes even prickling sensation that runs all the way down the leg.
- Numbness or weakness while walking or while moving the foot or leg.
- Shooting or severe pain that occurs usually in one leg and makes walking or standing up very difficult.
- Depending on the spot where the sciatic nerve is pinched or affected, the pain and other sciatica symptoms could also lead to pain in the toes and foot.

Even a single symptom could signify your condition of sciatica while some of you might have to wait for a combination of the symptoms. In any case, one should watch out for all these symptoms to confirm the sciatica condition.

Sciatica Symptoms for Each Nerve Root

As mentioned earlier, there are 5 root nerves in total. Two of these roots exit the lumbar spine (L4 and L5) and the remaining three exit the sacral segment (S1, S2, and S3).

All of these nerves combine together to form the large sciatic nerve. These nerves branch out again once they reach the leg to deliver sensory and motor functions to specific destinations in the foot and leg.

Sciatica symptoms greatly vary and depend on the region where the nerve root is pinched or suffocated. The location plays an important role in where you will feel the pain or other symptoms or sciatica pain. For instance, these are some of the symptoms related to the specific nerves.

L4 Nerve Root Sciatica

Symptoms related to this specific nerve usually have an impact on one of the thighs. Patients may feel weakness and pain in straightening the leg. This could cause them a trouble in walking and standing up after sitting. Patients may also have a diminished knee-jerk reflex.

L5 Nerve Root Sciatica

The symptoms for L5 nerve root sciatica pain may extend to the ankle as well as to the big toe. This symptom is also known as foot drop. Patients may experience feel numbness or pain on the top part of the foot, especially the part that is known as the 'web' of the skin that is exactly located between the big toe and second toe. The patient might also feel an uncomfortable sensation in their lower back.

S1 Nerve Root Sciatica

The symptoms of this particular nerve root affect the outer area of the foot. The pain, however, may radiate to all the toes. Patients who have their S1 nerve affected or pinched may also experience symptoms including weakness when lifting the foot from the ground or while standing on tiptoes. The payment may also experience reduction in the ankle-jerk reflex.

Bottom Line

It is not necessary for one patient to experience only one of the symptoms mentioned above. Since a patient may get one or more nerve roots compressed at a time, it is possible to experience multiple or a combination of symptoms from the ones listed above.

What Does the Doctor Say

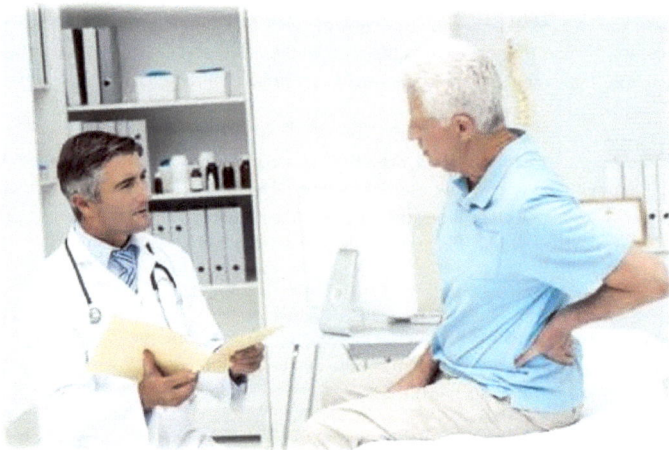

While some of the symptoms can be dealt with at home, as majority of the symptoms do not worsen quickly, some symptoms can become unbearable and may require immediate medical attention and even immediate surgery in some cases. The following are some of these symptoms that should be taken to the doctor:

1. Symptoms that progressively becomes worse instead of improving. This is when the pain might indicate towards nerve damage. This becomes especially very serious when the progressive symptoms are also very neurological –such as feeling of weakness in the back of the thigh and leg.
2. While majority of the symptoms are only associated with one leg, symptoms are often considered serious when they can be felt in both legs – also known as bilateral sciatica – and cause bowel or bladder dysfunction or incontinence. This may further lead to cauda equine syndrome. This particular syndrome is an acute compression associated with one or a combination of nerve roots that occur in very rare cases.

In both of these cases, patients should stop considering home remedies and other non-medical or alternative treatments and should immediately seek assistance from the doctor.

Bottom Line

Symptoms are the first indication of sciatica pain. If you are experiencing or a combination of these symptoms, go ahead and learn about your treatment options – both non-medical and medical-related and learn how you can take care of your sciatica pain.

Chapter 4 –Sciatica Treatment

For unbearable or continuous flare-up of sciatic nerve pain, the sciatica condition must be treated so that it does not progress or get worse with time.

Fortunately, for majority of the patients, regular exercise routine and readily available nonsurgical remedies can really help you get rid of the pain on a long-term basis. However, it is highly advisable that you seek permission from your doctor or take advice on the exercises or other alternative treatment before you start considering your options.

On the other hand, for patients who experience severe sciatica symptoms or pain, which continues to progress with time, it is important to take a more structured approach towards treatment. This could also include surgery as a possible option and in some cases, surgery is the only way to find long-term pain relieve as well as prevention from future dysfunction or pain.

But before we learn about sciatica surgery options, let's first learn about the non-surgical treatment options you have in hand. If your symptoms are mild, these treatments may come in handy for long-term benefits.

Non-Surgical Treatment for Sciatica

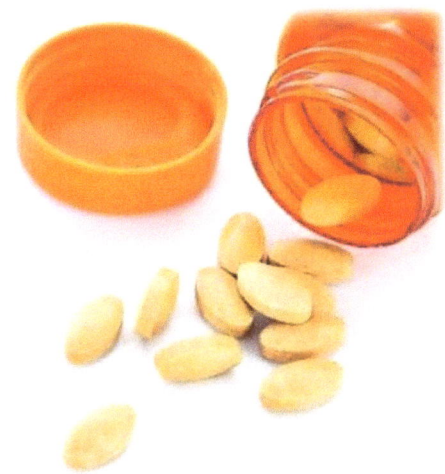

The main aim behind the non-surgical treatment options is to relieve sciatica pain as well as minimize neurological symptoms that are caused by choked nerve root. There are a number of options available when it comes to treating sciatica pain without surgery. All of these treatment options are covered in this chapter. Using one or a combination of the treatment mentioned in this chapter can help you go a long with sciatica pain. However, experts also suggest that following these alternative treatment methods along with indulging into some stretching exercises is an ideal way to achieve your goal.

Check out your non-surgical treatment options below.

Heating and Icing Therapies

Two of the most readily available treatments to relieve acute sciatic pain include the heating and icing therapies. These two methods are commonly used to alleviate lower back and leg pain, especially if the pain is in the first stage.

Icing and heating therapies are used multiple times in a day for effective results. While some people find more relief from the icing therapy, others find heating therapy more useful. The best part is, you do not have to choose between the two. In fact, you can alternate both the therapies to get better results.

But why is heating and icing beneficial for sciatica pain relief. Read on to find out more:

Heating Therapy

While the heat and warmth have always been associated with relaxation and comfort, when you specifically talk about heath therapy, the results and benefits go one step further and can provide you healing benefits as well as relief from pain. Heat therapies are extremely successful and beneficial when it comes to treating back pain, like sciatica.

Heating therapy can be provided in various ways. Heat therapy in the form of heat wraps, heating pads, warm gel packs, and hot baths are all great, easy and inexpensive ways to find relief from pain.

- **How Heat Therapy Works?**

The application of heat therapy can help provide lower back pain relief through a number of mechanisms, such as:

1. Heat therapy is considered beneficial because this one method helps dilate the blood vessels of the muscles that are around the lumbar spine region. This process is great for increasing the flow of nutrients and oxygen to the muscles, which also helps in healing the damaged tissue.
2. Heating also helps in stimulating sensory receptors present in the skin. This means that when you apply heat to your lower back or affected area, the signals of pain transmission to the brain will reduce and will help you feel comfortable.
3. The application of heat also facilitates making the soft tissues more stretchable around the lumbar spine, including adhesions, connective tissues, and muscles. Heat therapy helps calm down stiffness and improves overall flexibility to make you feel comfortable.

For most people, this inexpensive treatment works best when combined with other non-surgical treatments for sciatica pain, such as exercise and other physical therapies. Also, it is one of the most common therapies considered by patients because it is a non-pharmaceutical and non-invasive form of relieving lower back/sciatica pain.

- **How To Apply Heat Therapy**

Using heat therapy products is a simple way to provide adequate heat to the affected area for pain relief. However, it is important that you choose the therapy products wisely. Whatever you are using, make sure it can effectively maintain heat at the right temperature.

As far as the duration is concerned, the longer you can apply the heat, the better. However, for sciatica pain, it is recommended that you take the heating therapy for at least 20 minutes. In case the pain is too intense, longer heating therapy sessions can be more beneficial.

The following are two heat therapy methods:

1. **Dry Heat Therapy:** include options such as saunas and heating pads. While these are beneficial when it comes to relieving pain, this method also draws out moisture from the body and can leave your skin feeling dry and dehydrated. However, people still opt for this option as the results are great and it is easier to apply.
2. **Moist Heat Therapy:** include options such as hot baths, moist heating packs, or steamed towels. This method is also considered effective as it helps the heat to penetrate deep down in the muscles. The results are quicker and long-term in this case and therefore, most people choose this method for better pain relief.

Individuality is a very important factor here that should not be ignored. A therapy that might be successful for one person may not be suitable for another. So try experimenting with different methods to find out the one that works best for you.

Some common options for heating therapy include:

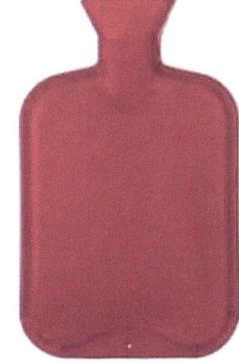

1. **Hot Water Bottle** –the bottle heating method has been around since forever. It is an effective tool since it tends to stay warm for up to 30 minutes. The heating is mild and perfect for relieving sciatica pain.
2. **Heated Gel Pad** – readily available, gel pads can be microwaved or heated in boiling water. These are also effective and can stay warm for 20-30 minutes.
3. **Electric Heating Pad** –is also great for maintaining a constant level of heat for as long it is plugged.
4. **Heat Wraps** –this method is ideal for low intensity of heat. The wraps can be easily wrapped around the waist and lower back area and can be worn under clothing. The method is convenient and provides long hours of heating application.
5. **Steam Bath, Sauna, Hot Tub, Hot Bath** –all of these moist heating methods are considered effective as they naturally stimulate general feelings of relaxation and comfort and may also reduce pain and muscle spasm.

Last but not the least, it is important to keep in mind that there's enough insulation between the skin and the heat source to avoid burning or overheating the skin.

- **When Heat Therapy Should Not Be Used**

Heat therapy should not be used without consent from your medical practitioner, especially if you are diagnosed with any medical condition. For instance, if you have bruised or swollen lower back, heating therapy is not recommended.

Patient should also see their doctors if they have hypertension or heart disease. The following are some conditions where heating therapy is not suitable:

- Deep vein thrombosis
- Dermatitis
- Peripheral vascular disease
- Diabetes
- Severe cognitive impairment
- Open wound

Generally, in case of an injury, bruise or swelling, it is better to use the icing therapy instead of heating. Read on to learn more about icing therapy and how it can help you relieve pain from sciatica condition.

Icing therapy

On the other hand, you have icing therapy as your option. While this method is completely opposite to that of heating therapy, the aim behind each therapy is the same – relief from pain.

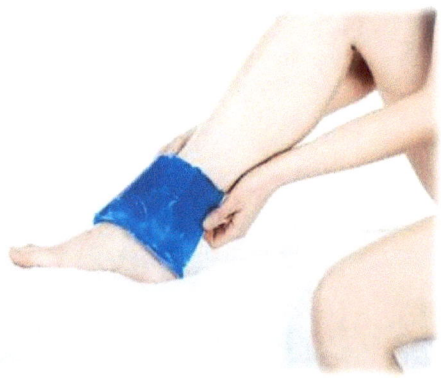

Ice therapy, just like heat therapy, is a convenient way to get rid of sciatica pain. The results might be temporary, but these methods help alleviate the uncomfortable pain and hurdles that come with sciatica pain. Simple application of ice or cold pack on the affected area (with a protective barrier between the pack and the skin to keep it from ice burn) is a very effective treatment available for pain relief.

Cold pack or ice wrapped in a tower or plastic bag can be applied on the affected area – your lower back, buttock or even thighs –several times in a day for desirable results. However, when dealing with the icing therapy, it is important to remember that the therapy should not exceed 20 minutes of time.

- **What Are the Different Types of Cold and Ice Packs?**

There are many different types of ice packs available that can be used for the therapy to relief lower back sciatica pain. All of the options covered here are effective in their own unique way. Again,it is important that you experiment with a few options to find out which option works best for you. Your choice will depend on budget, personal preference, as well as your convenience.

Some of the most common types of cold pack options available for your sciatica pain relief are as follows:

1. **Reusable Ice Pack or Cold Pack:** you can find different reusable ice packs readily available at general stores and drug stores. These packs are usually filled with gel. For the therapy, these packs are kept in the freezer until chilled and can be used whenever needed. The best part about these packs is that it can be reused time and again.

2. **Homemade Ice Pack:** if you are looking for cheaper options, you can even consider making ice pack at home. All you have to do is just grab some ice from your freezer and squeeze out the air from the bag and seal it up. Some people also prefer adding some chilled water to the bag to keep the bag from becoming lumpy. It is also important to create a barrier between the ice pack and your skin to make sure it does cause you ice burn. Thus, wrapping it up in a towel is a feasible option. Other alternatives for homemade ice pack include:
   a. **Sponge:** soak a sponge until wet and place it in the freezer. Once it is frozen, put the sponge in a baggier and seal. Then wrap it in a small tower or a thick sock before applying it to the affected area.
   b. **A Frozen Towel:** to prepare your towel cold pack, damp the towel and place it in a plastic bag. Put the bag into the freezer for 20 minutes and pull out the chilled towel from the bag. Wrap it around the affected area for relief in pain.
   c. **Rice:** grab a clean, washed sock and fill it with rice. Wrap it in the end and place it in the freezer until the rice is frozen. The best part about this method is that the rice is as chilled as ice and does not even melt during the therapy.
   d. **Frozen Bag of Peas:** This works exactly like rice. Just grab the packet of frozen peas or other vegetables, wrap it up in a thin towel and apply to the affected area for relief.

3. **Instant/Disposable Ice Packs:** One of the main reasons people opt for the reusable or homemade ones is because the instant or disposal ice packs are only for one time usage and therefore can be expensive. However, the advantages are big too. For instance, they are readily available and do not require the preparation or freezing time. They are instantly ready as soon as they are cracked due to a chemical reaction. Also, the chemical reaction helps the pack to keep cold for longer as compared to other methods. A variety of instant, disposable ice packs are available at most general merchandise and drug stores.

- **The Right Way to Use Ice Packs**

The following is a guide to ice massage therapy to get rid of sciatica pain. Following the method thoroughly will help you achieve optimal results:

1. The therapy should always be carried out in a circular motion and with gentle pressure only.
2. It is best to keep within the 6-inch range of the pain for the ice massage therapy to work best.
3. Ice massage should never be directly applied to the bony structure of the back. This is especially true for sciatica pain.
4. Ice massage should not be applied for more than 5 minutes in a go. Take a break and apply again and do that multiple times in a day for great results.
5. Repeat the ice massage a few times in a day.

- **Precautions to Take When Using Ice Packs**

In addition to the dos, it is also important that you are well aware of the don'ts of ice massage therapy. Here are some precautions you should keep in mind:

1. As mentioned a few times earlier, ice should never be applied directly on the skin. Creating a protective barrier – such as a towel – is very important to keep the skin from ice burn.
2. While the total duration of the ice massage therapy should now exceed 20 minutes, it is important to take breaks after every 5 minutes to avoid burning.
3. Ice patients is not recommended for patients diagnosed with other medical conditions, such as patients who have cold allergic conditions, areas of impaired sensation, paralysis, Raynaud's Syndrome and Rheumatoid arthritis.
4. Make sure you never fall asleep with ice pack resting on your skin.

Bottom Line

Icing therapy is considered the better option for instant relief. So follow the method carefully to gain benefit from these therapies to get rid of sciatica pain. However, even though both icing and heating options work, they are temporary and you would only be able to get rid of the pain for a while. Also, you cannot have access to heating and ice packs all the time and especially when you are work. Thus, sitting and working in constant pain can become unbearable. With sciatica, it is also important to maintain good spine posture, which is only possible if you have a good seating arrangement.

This is where Bael Wellness Sea Cushion comes in. As mentioned earlier, these cushions are ideal for people suffering through sciatica, orthopedic, coccyx and back and tailbone pain. It is specifically designed to help you keep your posture right and to prevent the pain. This could be your ultimate solution if you have to stir for prolong hours at work because it is made from Grade A memory foam with wedges and contours.

Just grab it with the build-in handle this seat cushion becomes portable. Carry it to work for your office seat, just place it on your car seat while you are driving, or place it on the chair while you are reading or dining at home. You can carry it where you go and can sit on this cushion to avoid back pain successfully.

Pain Medications

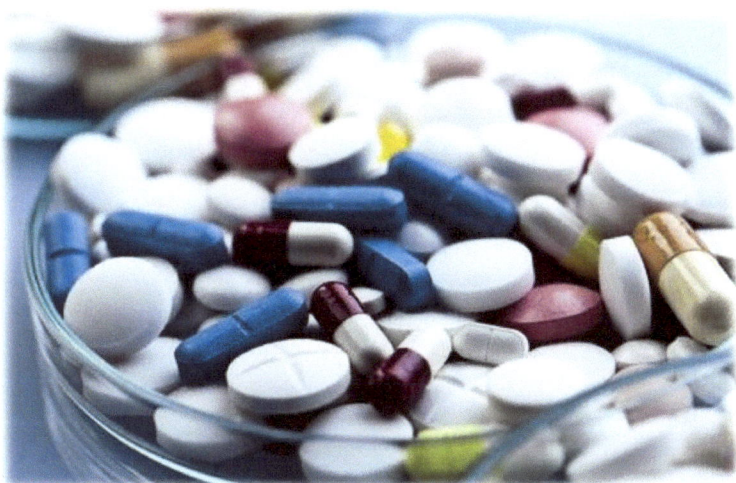

Prescription or over-the-counter medications are another option for relieving sciatica pain. These medicines are easily available and can be taken to reduce or control pain for a certain period. Non-steroidal anti-inflammatory drugs (such as naproxen, ibuprofen, or COX-2 inhibitors) are great for controlling inflammation.

Other than that, oral steroids can also be taken for reducing the level of inflammation which causes increased pain and severe symptoms in some cases.

NSAIDs is a whole class of drugs that comes with different options. Other than aspirin, there are currently a number of different types of non-prescription and prescriptions brands of NSAIDs available over the counter. However, the three most common types that are often suggested will include:

- **Naproxen (E.g. Naprosyn, Aleve)**
- **Ibuprofen (E.g. Nuprin, Motrin, Advil)**
- **COX-2 Inhibitors (E.g. Celebrex)**

While some of the pain killers can be taken without consulting the doctor, if you are diagnosed with any other medical problem or if you are not sure about your sciatica pain or if taking any of the above medication causes you discomfort or increase in pain, you should immediately seek assistance from a doctor. Also, medicines should only be considered if the symptoms of sciatica pain are increasing overtime.

Epidural Steroid Injections for Relieving Sciatica Pain

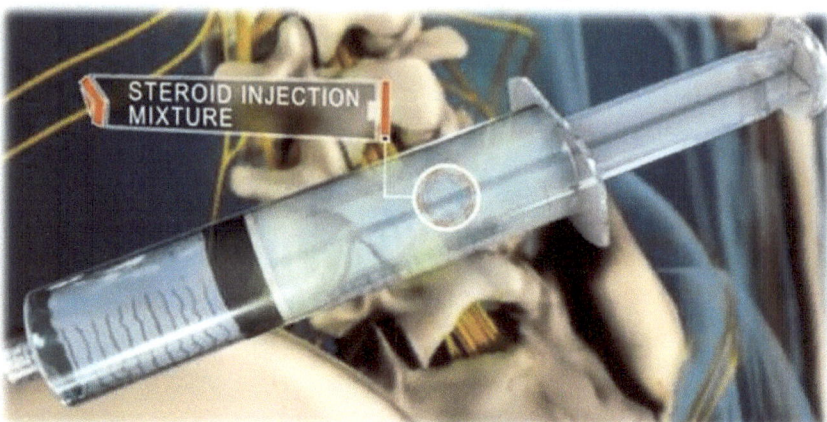

As far as sciatica treatment is concerned, epidural steroid injections are considered a minimally invasive option. In case the pain or other sciatica symptoms become severe, an epidural steroid injection can be taken for reducing the level of inflammation.

It is also important to learn that epidural injections work differently from oral medications. This is mainly because the epidural is directly injected into the area around the sciatic nerve and can instantly help reduce pain by decreasing the level of inflammation that could be the main culprit behind the sciatic pain sessions.

While the effects of epidural steroid injections are also temporary – just like oral medication, and can provide relief from pain to up to a year, these may not work for everyone. However, it is suitable for some people and can be very effective in relieving acute sciatic pain. More importantly, the relief from epidural steroid injections for sciatica can be sufficient enough to allow a patient to progress with exercise and other conditioning and yoga exercises.

The most positive point about these injections is that they deliver medication directly or very near to the affected area or the area where the pain is generating. On the other hand, painkillers and oral steroid have a less-focused, dispersed impact and may even cause unwanted side effects.

Moreover, since it is believed that majority of the symptoms and pain related to sciatica is caused by chemical inflammation, taking epidural steroid injections can even help control that and reduce the level of inflammation by flushing out inflammatory chemicals and proteins from the system, which further helps in relieving the pain.

Again, it is best to consider assistance from your doctor before taking the final decision.

Alternative Treatment Methods to Relieve Sciatica Pain

It is ideal to learn about all the options you have in hand before choosing for the right one. Fortunately, medication and injections aren't the only help you have for sciatica pain relief. In fact, there's a list of alternative treatment for sciatica that should be considered to improve your pain and overall condition.

Therefore, in addition to the medical treatments – both oral medication and epidural injection –there are a number of alternative treatments for sciatica pain available that have shown effective results for many patients. Three most popular and common form of alternative sciatica treatment include massage therapy, acupuncture, and chiropractic manipulation.

Learn about each of these options in detail in this chapter.

Chiropractic/Manual Manipulation

Manual manipulation and spinal adjustments performed by properly trained and experienced health professionals –such as osteopathic physicians and chiropractors –can help you achieve better alignment of spinal column, which in return helps treating the underlying causes that leads to sciatic nerve pain. In short, in addition to reducing the sciatica pain itself, this specific alternate treatment is also great for the underlying cause.

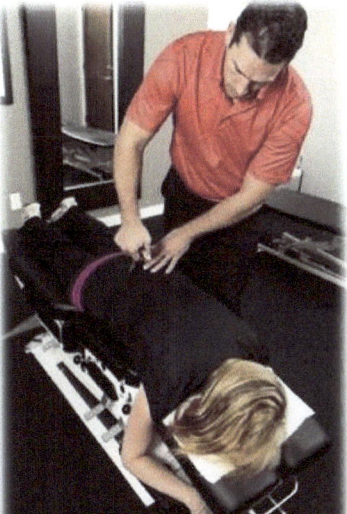

Make sure you only consider a professional chiropractor to carry out this method with you. Generally, these professionals have their special focus on treatment and manipulation of the spinal structure as well as the surrounding structures.

Since the method mainly focuses on the underlying causes, it is actually effective in relieving sciatica pain.

Alternative Chiropractic Treatment Core Purpose

The core purpose of considering this treatment method is to get rid of the sciatica pain and other symptoms as well as treat other common lower back pain conditions with the help of manual therapy.

- **Manual Manipulation and Spinal Manipulation:** This manipulation method refers to the short lever arm thrust applied to the abnormal vertebra with high velocity with the purpose of improving the alignment as well as the functionality. The trick also helps in restoring range of painless motion as well as nerve irritability in the lower back region. This practice is also commonly called 'chiropractic adjustment'.

- **Mobilization:** This technique refers to low velocity manipulation – unlike the manual or spinal manipulation –and revolves around stretching and movement of joints and muscles, with the goal of reducing pain and increasing normal motion ranges within the affected areas.

What is Chiropractic Adjustment Description?

A chiropractic adjustment is commonly known as manual manipulation, chiropractic manipulation, or spinal manipulation. All of these names suggest the same thing – the chiropractic therapy. It is a therapeutic treatment to help you say good-bye to your lower back pain by adjusting the spine and other structures.

The main objective behind this treatment is to reduce pain, reduce subluxation, with goals of improving overall function of the spine, as well as reducing nerve irritability and increasing the range of motion. Typically, chiropractic adjusts description involves the following:

- A short lever arm thrust is applied to the spine (mainly the vertebra) with high velocity to adjust the alignment and reduce lower back pain.
- An audible, accompanying release of gas this usually caused by the release of carbon dioxide, nitrogen, and oxygen, which as a combination releases cavitation (joint pressure).
- While the immediate effect often leads to short-term discomfort, patients report great relieve in pain and better motion sensation. The pain or minor discomfort is often caused by spasm or tense up in muscles during the procedure.

All in all, it is very important that you choose the right chiropractor, who's both professional and skilled to ensure you will actually say good-bye to your sciatica pain.

Acupuncture

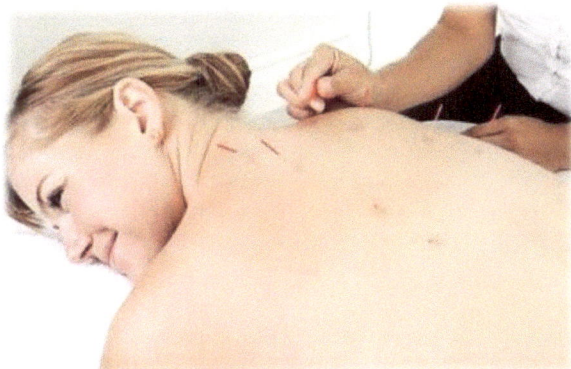

Acupuncture no longer requires an introduction. The technique has become so popular lately, that everyone's well aware about the procedure as well as the benefits associated with it. It is widely known and accepted as an alternative, non-traditional treatment, which can be used to relieve neck and back pain, successfully.

While acupuncture is not the first alternative treatment that is considered to sought neck and back problems, more and more sciatica patients are turning towards this treatment for successful results. This alternative therapy is successful can also be judged by the fact that not only patients, even health professionals including physicians are starting to use acupuncture to fight off their back and neck pain. The treatment has similar amazing benefit for treating sciatica pain as well.

Acupuncture can be traced back to 2500 years ago in the form of Chinese medical therapy. The theory of acupuncture says that our body has 2000 points that are associated with 20 pathways, commonly known as meridians. These pathways help the life force or vital energy of the body – which is referred to as qi –flows throughout the body. Acupuncture therapy requires lots of hair-thin needles to be inserted into those points in unique combinations in order to correct or maintain the right flow of qi (pronounced as chee).

How Does Acupuncture Works?

It is believed that the effects come from stimulating the central nervous system. This procedure helps release the chemicals into the muscles, brain, as well as spinal cord. These chemicals are either responsible to alter how pain feel like or produce internal physical changes that promotes the sense of well-being.

There are other theories associated with acupuncture that may suggest something totally different. Other theories suggest that this alternative Chinese therapy works by:

1. The insertion of thin needles speed up the relay of electro-magnetic signals. This is the point where the chemicals with pain killing properties are generated. Such chemicals are also known as endorphins. The flow of these chemicals helps alleviate pain and give you comfort.
2. The insertion of needles is also believed to release immune system cells that enhance the overall well-being of the body and thus helps alleviate pain and other uncomfortable symptoms.
3. The procedure may also trigger the release of natural opioids. Again, these are natural chemicals present in the brain that promote sleepiness and reduce the intensity of pain.
4. The procedure may also change the chemistry of your brain by changing the release of neurohormones and neurotransmitters. The latter are responsible for either dampening the nerve impulse or stimulating it. Neurohormones can also have an impact on the activity or function of different organs in your system.

Since the therapy requires the usage of multiple needs and the right understanding of certain points out of the 2000 points in our body, it is essential that you only consult an experienced professional. It is indeed recommended that you consider alternative treatment therapy to find relief in pain and other symptoms of sciatica pain.

Massage Therapy

Many sciatica patients turn to different massage therapies to reduce their lower back pain and feel better. Indeed, there are different types of therapies that result in a number of great benefits in helping the patients alleviate back pain.

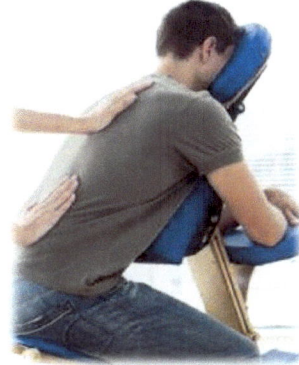

Massage therapy for your back pain is believed to have a number of benefits, including muscle relaxation, improved blood circulation, and release of natural pain relieving chemicals known as endorphins. It is the benefits that have helped massage therapy to evolve so much and become popular amongst patients who constantly suffer back pain. According to a survey, the number of patients of adults receiving massage therapy is doubling after every decade from 1997.

A number of healthcare providers consider massage therapy as the ultimate solution for lower back pain. In fact, more than 50% of healthcare professionals admit that they will encourage patients to get massage treatment along with taking their respective medical treatment for better results.

Benefits of Massage Therapy for Sciatica Pain

According to a research conducted by the American Massage Therapy Association, there are a number of important health benefits, including relieve in lower back pain that is associated with massage therapy. Some of these benefits are listed below:

- **Improved Blood Circulation:** Blood circulation is important for our entire system. Massage therapy helps the blood circulation to improve which helps in recovery of muscle soreness from physical activity.
- **Muscle Relaxation:** Since sciatica pain can also affect the muscle and tighten it up – especially the major thigh muscle – massage helps the muscles to relax and become flexible again. The muscle relaxation can also help you with insomnia.
- **Improved Range of Motion:** Again, stiff and sore muscles can affect your range of motion. Once your pain is under control and your muscles are flexible again, it is easier for you to move and indulge into a range of motions and physical activities.
- **Increased Levels of Endorphins:** Massage therapy also helps our brain to produce more endorphins. This is actually one of the best benefits you can gain from massage therapy. The production and increased level of this natural chemical in the body ensures your well-being. Endorphins reduce the intensity of pain and help you feel good on the whole. It is also very effective for managing chronic pain.

Even if you are taking any medication, massage therapy can be the additional treatment for greater results and benefits.

Treatment Methods for Recurring Sciatica Pain

For most people, sciatica is a condition that can better on its own or with little non-surgical treatment. However, the healing process for some people may take up to weeks. But in the end, most people do not really require medical attention to treat their sciatica pain or other symptoms.

Overall, the different and episodes of sciatica pain gets better within a period of six to twelve weeks. While medication can be your first priority when it comes to relieving initial pain, you can even consider a program of exercise or physical therapy to minimize the symptoms as well as the pain associated with sciatica.

Exercise, especially the stretching poses, is great for naturally treating your sciatica pain. That is covered in more detail in the next chapter. For now, all you have to focus on is to connect with a spine care professional, who specializes in taking care of sciatica symptoms. These spine care professionals may include physiatrists (rehabilitation and physical medicine specialist), chiropractors, physical therapists, and pain medicine specialist. These professional people are trained not only to provide relief from pain but also help prevent the recurrences of sciatica in future.

The only thing you need to keep in mind is to consult only a qualified medical professional to take care of your sciatica symptoms and provide you treatment.

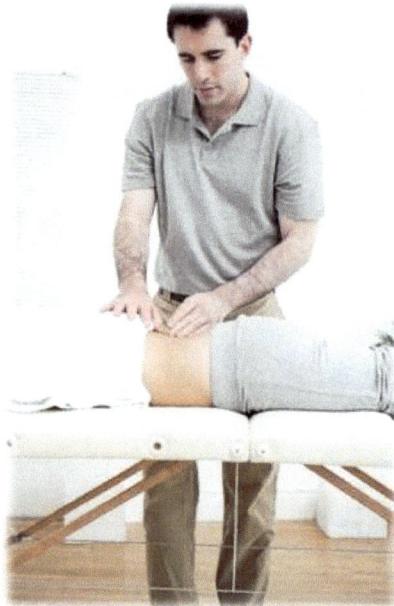

Chapter 5 – Sciatica Pain Relief Exercises

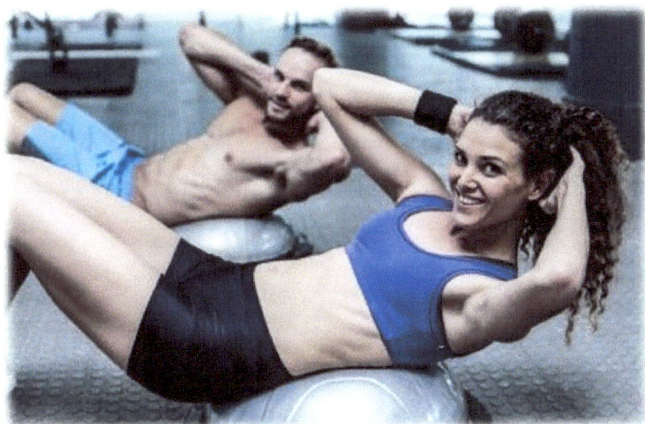

As mentioned earlier a few times, exercise plays an important role in keeping your spine healthy. A healthy spine does not ache or show any other sciatica symptoms. If you have not paid attention to this earlier, now is the time to indulge into physical activities and exercise programs to relief sciatica pain.

For majority instances related to sciatica pain, it is important to create a progressive, controlled, and specific exercise program that is designed to address the underlying cause that leads to sciatica pain. If the symptoms are mild, you can get into little movement or exercise that suits you. However, if your case is serious and the pain is getting worse, it is ideal to consider a medical professional to design an exercise program for you that treats your underlying condition.

The specific exercises recommended for sciatica serves two main purposes:

1. Reduces pain and other symptoms associated with sciatica in the near term.
2. Provides overall condition to our body that helps prevent sciatica pain in future and also offers us other benefits of staying fit – such as reduced risk of diabetes, obesity, and other heart diseases.

The right people to consult include a chiropractor, therapist, certified athletic trainer, physiatrist (Physical Medicine and Rehabilitation Physician), and other spine specialists who are known for treating different sciatica symptoms and pain. Get your program designed according to your needs and let the professional teach you how to perform these exercises.

Go through this chapter and learn more about the role of exercise for treating sciatica pain.

How Exercise Provides Relief in Sciatica Pain

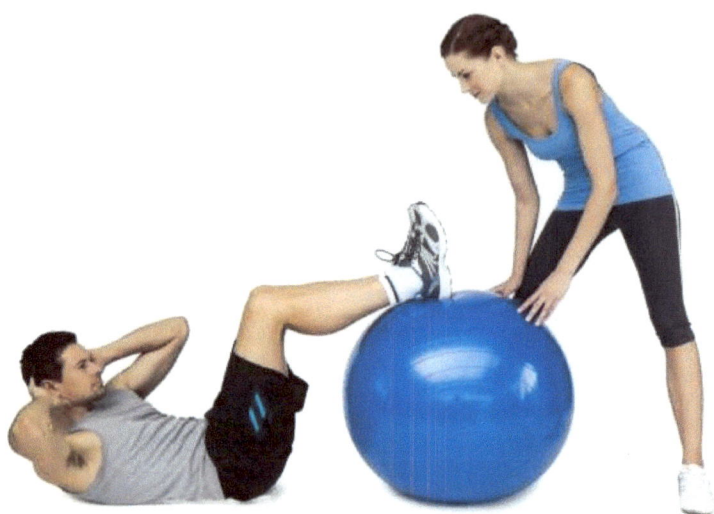

While this may come as a surprise to you, but exercise and regular physical activity is much better for relieving sciatic pain as compared to resting. While you feel comfortable while you are on bed, it isn't treating your condition. It is just a temporary relief and the pain will come back crawling as soon as you get up. Also, going on a bed rest may further stiffen your muscles and cause you trouble in moving or walking.

In case the pain flares up and become really intense, you may rest for a day or two, but if you continue to take bed rest, the inactivity will only make your pain worse.

It is common for your spinal structures as well as muscles to become de-conditioned due to lack of movement and exercise. This can further lead to strain and back injury if not taken care of properly. In short, if you want to get rid of the pain, you have to push yourself and get yourself moving, despite the pain. Once your structure becomes used to the exercise routine, you will notice improvement in your flexibility.

Additionally, active exercises also helps in exchanging fluids and nutrients within the spine and disc are to keep the pressure from forming on the sciatic nerve as well as to keep the discs healthy. So before you consult any professional, it is important that you have a clear understanding of the typical features associated with sciatica exercise program. All of this is covered in detail this chapter, so keep reading.

Core Muscle Strength

Majority of the exercises suggested for sciatica treatment will serve to strengthen the back and abdominal muscles in order to provide proper support for the back. Strengthening exercises that targets the core muscles may first seem difficult to perform and may even cause pain since the muscles are inflexible and tight and you are already experiencing sciatica pain.

However, when you regularly indulge in the exercise program, and push your harder each time, you will start seeing the benefits of stretching and strengthening exercises for your core muscles. Regular exercise will help you alleviate sciatica pain and recover quickly from other symptoms and will also reduce chances of future sciatica pain episodes.

The following are two most popular and effective core exercises that you can perform at home. Follow the instructions and seek assistance from a professional if you are not able to do it yourself.

- **Circle Plank**

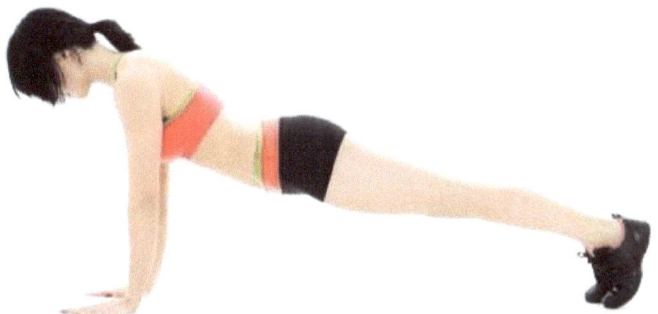

Start with your regular plank position, facing downwards with both your elbows straight and palms touching the ground and your body stretching out straight with your lower body weight on your toes. Keep your body straight and get into the right posture to avoid causing more pain.

Bend your right leg and pull your knee closer to your chest. All your body weight will shift to your right toes. Start moving your right knee in circle in a clockwise direction once. Complete another circle in an anticlockwise direction. Make sure the rest of your body is in stationary position. Repeat the clockwise and anticlockwise circles fives time with your right knee. Switch legs and continue the same way.

At first you may not be able to hold on for too long, especially due to sciatica pain. However, try to increase the repetition and circles with each routine to gain better results. Last but not the least, just pay attention to your posture and make sure your back is straight at all times.

- **Forward Bend**

This traditional and simple exercise can help you go a long way in keeping sciatica pain at bay. This is a simple exercise but it is important to be conscious about your posture to avoid the pain from getting worse.

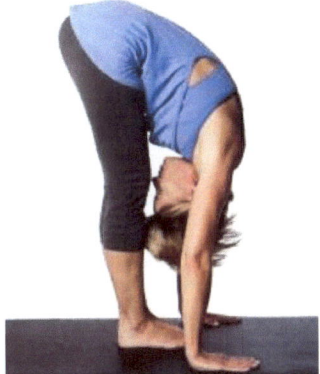

To perform this one, just stand straight with your feet close to each other and your shoulder straight. Raise your arms above your head with your elbows stretched. Slowly start bending your back, inhale to stick your tummy in tight and try to touch floor if you can.

Again, it might be difficult for you to do this at first, but with regular practice and a little more effort each time, you will be able to do this without any trouble. Also, make sure you bring your neck down too as you bend forward and put your palms on the floor.

At this point, exhale and slowly move all the way up with your hands above your head. Do 10 reps and relax. You can also increase the reps with time for better and quicker results. Not only this exercise is great for strengthening core muscles but also helps alleviate sciatica pain, effectively.

You will learn about more exercises and postures later in this chapter.

Specific Diagnosis

In addition to understanding why core muscle exercises are important for sciatica pain treatment, it is also important to understand that specific diagnosis is crucial. It is advised that you take suggestions for your exercise program from a professional because in some cases, programs are designed to meet your specific requirements according to the underlying cause that causing you sciatic pain – such as spinal stenosis and lumbar herniated disc.

Indulging into the wrong exercises or doing them the wrong way can worsen the sciatic pain as well as the underlying condition. Thus, accurate diagnosis is essential prior to starting sciatica exercises. However, this book covers some of the most common and popular exercises that are generally suggested by the professionals. In case your body is not used to exercise or if you don't know how to perform certain exercises, it is best to leave it to the professionals as it is about a very sensitive part of your body – your spine.

Hamstring Stretching

While specific diagnosis is important, majority sciatica symptoms can treated or benefit from a regular, more general routine, which includes hamstring stretching exercises. The hamstrings are a major group of muscles located in the thigh area. Sciatica and its underlying causes often leads to tightening and stiffening of hamstring muscles, which eventually stress on the low back and cause pain.

Hamstring stretching exercises, which helps bring back flexibility to the muscles, can be a great way to alleviate sciatica pain. Two of the most popular hamstring stretching exercises that any sciatica patient can do include the following:

- **Tipover Tuck Stretch**

This stretch is not only great for your hamstring muscles but also helps you loosen tight shoulder muscles. To perform this exercise, stand with your feet shoulder-width distance apart. Move you're your hands behind your back and hold in a tight grip. Start bending forward with your face moving towards the ground but keeping your knees straight. Tuck your chin tight and bend as much as you can as you stretch your arms and raise them above your head as much as possible.

You should feel the muscles being stretched out. However, if the stretch is too intense or if it is causing your pain or discomfort, release your hands and place them on the back of your thighs instead. Also, you can soften your knees to make the stretch easier for you. Hold this posture for 30 seconds and roll back to the initial position slowly.

- **Standing Hamstring Stretch**

This is a very simple stretch that offers great results. Even though the stretch isn't that deep here, this variation will surely help you avoid sciatica pain and other symptoms successfully. It is best to perform this stretch exercise after a run on your treadmill or in the part. This already warm up your muscles and it stretching will make them more flexible easily.

You will need a thigh high table to perform this exercise. Place the table right in from of you and stand at your leg distance. Now lift up your right leg and place the heel on the surface of the table. The surface will be slightly lower than your hip and will create the perfect posture for this exercise. Keep your foot flexed and feel the stretch in your calves, the back of your thighs and your buttock.

To increase the stretch, place your hands on top of your right thigh and bend forward towards your foot, by creasing at your hips. Hold that posture for 30 seconds and switch to the left leg.

There are other hamstring stretch exercises too. Don't forget to check with your healthcare professional before adding the others to your exercise program.

Correct Way of Exercising

As an addition to the hamstring muscle point, the correct way of exercising is as important as doing the right exercises. For instance, if you have chosen the best exercises for your sciatica pain relieve exercise program, but failing to do them correctly can make the program ineffective. In fact, in some cases, it can cause you more pain and problems than helping you get rid of them. In order to avoid increased or continued pain, it is very important that you follow the correct way of exercising.

If you haven't performed the exercises mentioned here or the ones outlined by your healthcare professional, it is best to do them under the supervision of your trained health practitioner – such as a physiatrist, chiropractor, physical therapist or a certified physical trainer.

Aerobic Exercises

Along with specific back pain exercises and stretches, aerobic conditioning is also encouraged for general fitness as well as to treat different underlying causes of sciatica pain. However, it is important to remember that low-impact aerobic exercises are best for sciatica patients because it comes with a number of benefits.

Aerobic Exercise Benefits for Sciatica Patients

Reconditioning done through low-impact aerobic exercises is useful for both maintenance and rehabilitation of the lower back region. Patients who are active and regularly indulge in aerobic exercises are less likely to experience severe sciatica symptoms as well as are able to condition their spine health in several ways. Here are some of benefits associated with aerobic exercise.

- Patients who regularly do aerobics experience fewer sciatica symptoms and episodes of back pain. They also experience less pain during an episode.
- Patients who actively participate in aerobic exercises stay more functional (carrying out their daily chores, recreational activities, and other work) as compared to patients who do not indulge into aerobic exercise. Other patients often end up losing functional capabilities in the long term.
- With aerobic exercise, it is easier for patients to lose or control weight, which is also essential for your spine health. Less weight means lesser stress on the joints and spinal structure.

- Aerobic is also one of the major contributors towards an increased production of endorphins. People who regularly perform aerobic exercises are in a better position to combat muscle and sciatica pain. These natural chemicals present in the body works as painkillers and thus helps a patient feel better.
- Endorphins released after an aerobic workout session can also help relieve symptoms of depression by elevating mood. Depression is a common side-effect of back injury or back pain.

Types of Low-Impact Aerobic Exercises for Sciatica Pain

It is ideal to consider low-impact aerobic exercises only because they are gentle on the back and does not cause more trouble. The following are some of these exercises that are extremely effective in providing conditioning to your spinal health.

- **Walking:** Whether on a treadmill or in a park in the open.
- **Bicycling:** Again, you can opt for a stationary bike at home or go for cycling outside. However, stationary bikes are recommended for patients who find standing more comfortable than sitting.
- **Step Machine or Elliptical Trainer:** These machines are effective and low-impact at the same time. The pedals help us move in a continuous manner which keeps our muscle moving.
- **Water Therapy:** If you enjoy swimming, it can really help you alleviate back pain.

Bottom Line

All of these factors discussed above can work as an effective treatment to take care of sciatica pain. It is important to keep these factors in mind, especially when talking to your healthcare professional to suggest you an exercise program. Make sure you discuss all the important points about your specific condition to get a custom-made program that is suitable for you.

Yoga for Sciatica – 4 Simple Moves to Ease Sciatica Pain

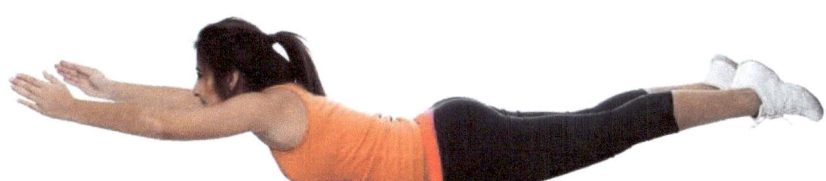

Talk about strengthening and stretching exercises for sciatica pain relief and you cannot leave behind yoga. Without a doubt, yoga is extremely beneficial for sciatica patients to minimize symptoms and to bring back the lost flexibility due to stiff muscles.

Yoga is most suitable in situations where your sciatica is caused by a bulging or herniated disk. Different yoga poses that progress from the gentles ones to foundational asanas will strengthen, lengthen, and align your lower back.

Start with doing all these moves at least three times in a week. Once you feel reduction in the pain, continue with the exercises at least once in a week to avoid recurrence of sciatica pain and symptoms. Here you will learn about the 4 most popular and effective yoga moves that will help you ease sciatica pain and make you functional again.

Reclining Cow's Face Pose

Cow's Face Pose is great to relieve sciatic tension by opening the muscles in the hips. This exercise is extremely beneficial for the type of sciatica that you get from very long hours of sitting. Desk jobs are the main reason why people have to sit in front of the computer for long hours. If that's the case with you, you can definitely try this exercise. Other than that, you can also use the Bael Wellness Seat Cushion that is especially designed for sciatica patients. In order to avoid the pain from coming back again and again, these cushions can be used as prevention.

Begin by lying on the ground on your back. Keep your knees bent and face up. Raise your left leg high and cross it over to place on the right one. Flex both feet and raise your right leg from the ground ultimately lifting the left one too. Bring it closer to your chest until your legs are hugging your belly. Spread your toes and keep your feet flex as your legs are crossed with each other. Hold your legs in this position for several breaths while you can feel the stretch in your legs as well as in your lower back. You can keep your hands on each leg to support the pose.

Release and let your feet rest on the ground again. Now switch legs and repeat to complete one set.

Low Lunge

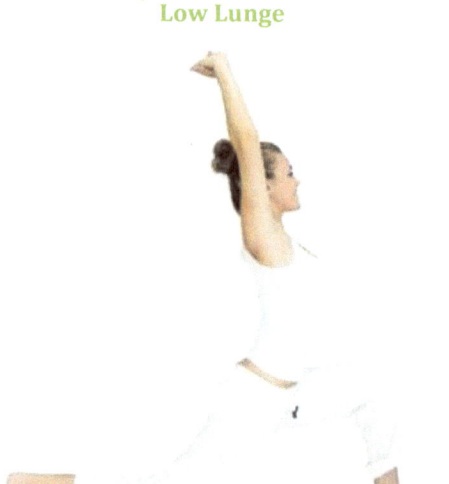

To see how this pose is performed, you can refer to the picture above. This pose targets several important muscles that will help you say good-bye to sciatica pain.

To begin with, get down on your yoga mat and start in a runner's lunge. Bend your right leg forward with knee over ankle and place your left knee on the ground with the top part of your foot touching the mat. Lift up your torso gradually and rest your hands on the right thigh. Make sure your right knee is behind toes at all times and lean your hips in a forward direction slightly. This way you will feel the stretch in the left hip flexor.

Stay in that posture for a while and to take this pose to the next level, raise your arms above your head with the biceps right next to your eat. Keep your hand close and in a forward stretch. Hold there for a while and repeat on the opposite side.

Raising your hand above your head will increase the intensity of the stretch. Therefore, you can practice that once you are in form and are able to take all that pressure on your back. Repeat with the other leg and complete set before moving on to the next pose.

Thread the Needle Pose

Lie on your back on the mat and keep both your knees bent. Lift up your left leg and place the ankle on the right knee. You will see a "4" shape designed with your legs. Put your left hand at the back of your right thigh from the space created in the center and clasp it with your right hand holding down from the right-hand side. Once your right knee is in your hands, lift up the right foot and bring it closer to your chest.

Make sure you keep both your feet in a flexed position throughout the posture. Bring it as close as you can to increase the stretch. Hold on for 30 seconds and release. Take your feet back to the ground in a gentle manner. Switch legs and repeat the pose to complete one set.

Pigeon Pose

Get into the runner's lunge once again with your right leg in front of you. Put your right knee over the ankle to get into the right pose and place your left knee on the ground with the top part of your left foot touching the mat. Bend your right food towards left and drop the thigh and shin to the floor. Make sure your knee is in line with your hip. Keep your left leg in the same but more relaxed form.

Stay in this posture for a while and allow your hips to get into the pose. Hold here or you can bend down from your torso and touch your forehead on your forearms. This will intensify the pose and will increase the stretch. Hold in that pose for around 30 seconds and release. Switch sides and repeat.

While performing this pose, you want to feel a moderate stretch in the outer side of the thigh. However, for people with severe sciatic pain, this pose can be a bit too challenging. If this one becomes too uncomfortable, you can stick to the Threat the Needle pose.

Bottom Line

Add these and other yoga poses to your exercise routine after consulting your healthcare professional and enjoy becoming functional again with more flexibility and without the obstacle of sciatic pain.

Chapter 6: Sciatica Surgery

While surgery is the last resort, for some people it is the only option available. Generally, the following are some situations in which considering surgery is valid:

1. Severe pain in the leg and in the lower back region that has persisted for longer than 4-6 weeks.
2. No results of pain relief are achieved after a constant effort of non-surgical sciatica treatments, such as one of multiple oral steroids, alternative therapies, medicines, and exercise.
3. The condition is becoming severe by the day and is limiting the patient's ability to carry out daily activities.

Urgent requirement of sciatic surgery is generally only important if the patient is progressively experiencing too much pain, weakness in the lower body, sudden loss of bladder or bowel control, and other severe symptoms.

On the basis of the duration and severity of the sciatica pain, two of the following procedures are considered:

Microdiscectomy for Sciatica

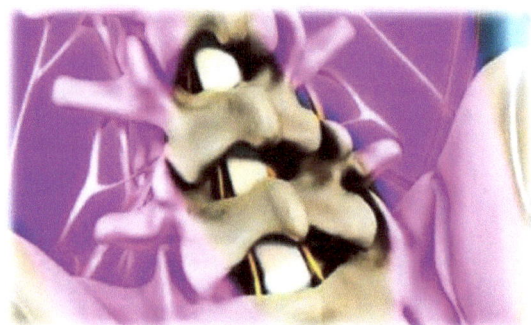

This option is often given to patients who are experiencing sciatic pain due to lumbar disc herniation. A microdiscectomy is often suggested to such patients. In this particular surgery, only the part of the herniated disc that is causing problem or that has pinched the sciatic nerve root is removed. The remaining disk remains intact.

This surgery is often suggested if the nerve pain does not diminish after 4-6 weeks and if multiple non-surgical methods have already been used without any results. If the pain is causing disability to the patient, surgery may not be considered sooner than the stated period.

Generally, more than 90 percent of the patients experience relief from their sciatica pain once this surgery is done.

Lumbar Laminectomy for Sciatica

On the other hand, sciatica that is caused by lumbar spinal stenosis, a lumbar laminectomy will be suggested to the patient. Similar to the previous one, this surgery will also involve removal of the disc or bone material that is irritating the sciatic nerve.

Laminectomy surgery is often given as an option for patients whose activity tolerance goes beyond the unacceptable level. That is like not in the functionality mode anymore.

However, before the final decision for the surgery is taken, it is important to take the general health of the patient into consideration as well. In this case, around 70 to 80 percent of patients experience relief from their sciatic nerve pain.

What's Patient's Decision?

In majority cases, surgery is often kept as a last resort and still is elective – which means that a patient may choose whether to have or not to have surgery. This is applicable for both types of surgeries mentioned above.

As far as the decision of the patient is concerned, it is mainly based on the severity of the symptoms, pain and dysfunction that patient is experiencing. Also, the duration of the condition will also play an important role whether or not to opt for surgery.

Doctors also consider the overall health condition of the patient before making surgery-related recommendations.

The Final Decision

Sciatica is a very subjective condition that varies from person to person – both in terms of severity and symptoms. What might be suitable for someone else may not be the right option for you. Thus, experimenting and experiencing is important. For that, you must keep the decision for surgery at the end of the list.

Start with your other options – medical non-surgical treatment, alternative therapies and exercise programs. Choose a combination of these to help you with your condition. Consider surgery only when everything else fails to work for you or if the condition gets worse instead of improving.

As far as experiencing and knowing all your options is concerned, you must not forget about Bael Wellness Seat Cushion either. It is definitely a great, portable solution that can help you get rid of pain and even improve your condition without non-surgical or surgical treatment. In fact, if you learn to keep your posture right simply by using a seat cushion and using it to sit – whether you are work, at a stadium enjoying a match or using your laptop or eating with family at home – you can say goodbye to back pain forever. Especially designed for people with sciatica, this option can definitely work wonders.

This book contains details about all your options as well as conditions so you find the most suitable treatment for yourself. Once you are able to diagnose your specific conditions following symptoms and other rules, you will be in a much better position to take a decision for your treatment as well.

So learn everything and start implementing now. Don't forget to seek assistance from a medical professional for best treatment and star t following the other tips and tricks that help you get rid of sciatica pain and other symptoms once and for all.

Use the information given in this book in your best interest and start your journey to live a pain-free life without sciatica again!

www.ingramcontent.com/pod-product-compliance
Lightning Source LLC
Chambersburg PA
CBHW050817290526
45792CB00001B/152